Herbal Remedies for Weight Loss and Wellness

All You Need to Know About Natural Remedies and Herbal Supplements to Restore Balance and Stimulate Natural Weight Loss

by Marta Tuchowska

Table of Contents

Introduction

Thank you for taking an interest in my book. It really means a lot to me. I am always very happy to share my passion for natural therapies with others. I have created this mini guide to introduce you to phytotherapy herbal treatments that you can use as an additional strategy in your weight loss efforts. If you are looking for natural solutions at affordable prices, then you have found your guide! If you have already achieved your ideal weight, some natural treatments that I recommend can help you maintain it as well as increase your energy levels, and as they say: keep on (*healthy)* track. Maybe you grabbed this book because you are really interested in natural therapies or are fascinated by phytotherapy(=herbalism) and healthy lifestyle and have made a vow to live even healthier. No matter what your reasons are, I welcome you all!

Before you start reading, I would like to make a mini disclaimer (I might be too repetitive with my disclaimers—sorry in advance!) about weight loss and fat burning supplements in general. As you may have noticed, the market is oversaturated with them. There are plenty of different so-called miracle *diet pills* or *weight loss supplements* that can be really detrimental to your health. My book does not recommend any of those. Moreover, many of those fad or fake supplements claim to be natural, and this is where the whole confusion starts. Many people don't trust the word *natural* anymore.

In my book, I talk about *real* natural phytotherapy supplements. Many naturopathic and therapeutic diets, like for example, The Alkaline Diet, The Paleo Diet, and the Macrobiotic Diet recommend herbal treatments as a part of getting back to our roots and stimulating our digestion.

I have also tried my best to include all necessary precautions that you should bear in mind before employing phytotherapy.

Something that is considered to be healthy, in general, can become unhealthy or even dangerous when abused. Too much of a good thing can become a bad thing. So please, do not treat this book as the ultimate solution. Weight loss is, in fact, a process that should be made as healthy as possible. The same applies to all kinds of cleanses that you may have chosen to do to restore your energy levels and even the *clarity of thought*. So first of all, be PATIENT! Rome wasn't built in a day. However, I am sure that this book will also encourage you to take action and add some new healthy habits to your life. The first results, like for example, feeling better in your body, will come sooner than you expect.

In this book, you will learn about:

-The best natural supplements to aid you in enhancing your metabolism, controlling appetite, and consuming fats for energy;

-The best energy revitalizing natural supplements that will support you throughout your strenuous physical activities and workouts;

-Natural teas and herbal infusions that deliver instant benefits to help you reach your weight goal faster;

-The benefits of natural, fresh juices and smoothies, and how they work for you; along with some great recipe tips and ideas.

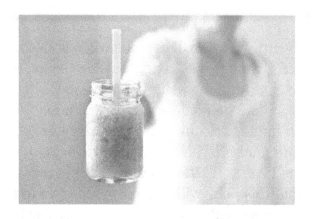

Of course, you need to remember that using natural food supplements alone is not the recommended way of losing weight; they should be used as a complement to get more successful results from a healthy and balanced diet and a regular physical exercise regime that you choose to do. If you are really determined to lose weight or keep your healthy weight, and are committed to it, ready to do whatever it takes, then natural remedies and food supplements will help to make your weight loss efforts more effective, faster, easier, as well as healthier.

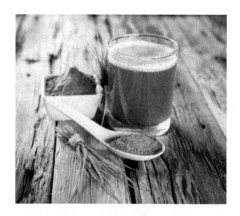

As I have already mentioned, there are many debates going on and some skepticism when it comes to magical weight loss pills. However, the solutions presented in this book are totally natural: Many phytotherapy plants can be taken in the form of capsules, tablets, as well as infusions. However, the first two modes are much easier to use, and many phytotherapists(=herbalists) I know say that they are even more powerful. Personally, I prefer to take my time and prepare a nice, herbal infusion, just like my Paleolithic ancestors! But I must admit that I also buy powdered herbs and very often add them to smoothies and my healthy desserts. Real time saver. The herbal powder that I mention, is what can be found inside those phytotherapy capsules (or tablets). Of course, if you want to be 100% natural, nothing can beat herbal infusions. If you are really busy, I would recommend using herbs in their powdered form (capsules and tablets). Always, <u>always research the brand</u>. The fact that a supplement is called: *natural*, does not mean that it actually is. There are many **harmful supplements** on the market that maybe do use some natural extracts, but most of them are pure chemicals, and you are never 100% sure what you are taking. So please—be careful. Use real **natural supplements** and real **phytotherapy**!

I have decided to create this book, to share my knowledge with you, and help make it as easy as possible for you to understand and apply. The methods described helped me improve my health and vitality, and if you give them a try, they can help you too. I also hope that they will help you become more energized as well as passionate about your healthy balance—something that is definitely worth working on hard.

How to use this guide?

As I have already said, I can't offer you the so-called ultimate solutions. I have prepared this mini guide for informative and introductory purposes. I have also shared my own experiences. I suggest you read through carefully, and pick up some of my suggestions that you think could work for you (keeping the precautions in mind—always!). The next step should be talking to your physician as well as to your herbalist (or naturopathic doctor). Do not self-medicate. Even with natural stuff! Herbs are more powerful than you think. Also, as they say: *different strokes for different folks*. For example, what worked for me might not for you, and what is great for you might make me sick. The same applies to different measurements; I believe that they cannot be prescribed equally for everyone reading the same book. This is why I have included a wide range of options.

3 Free eBooks

Thanks again for taking interest in my little book, I hope you will enjoy it, and that it will be able to help you discover something new and incredibly healthy as well.

I also have a free set of complimentary eBooks you can get by signing up to my health newsletter (free of charge):

www.HolisticWellnessProject/alkaline

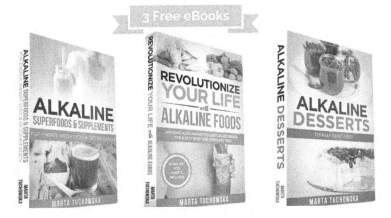

-They will show you a ton of healthy tips that you can apply to create a balanced lifestyle.

-They will also help you change your relationship with the concept of "dieting" or "calorie counting".

The best part? You will automatically join my **VIP Alkaline Wellness Newsletter** where I share the best of my tips, recipes and even motivational tools. You will also be notified about my new books when they are free or only 99c. Not **to mention killer bonuses** and insider news.

Don't worry about annoying marketing emails. I hate them as much as you do. The reason why I started a newsletter is to connect with my readers and help them with information, motivation, and inspiration they need for their body-mind transformations.

www.HolisticWellnessProject/alkaline

Congratulations for taking this very important step to take care of your body and mind in a holistic way! You will love it!

DISCLAIMER:

A physician has not written the information in this book. Although natural remedies are generally safe to use, if you suffer from a serious medical condition, are pregnant, or on medication, you should consult your physician first to check if it is safe to apply the natural remedies and food supplements described in this book. For prolonged treatments, it is also advisable that you visit a naturopathic doctor or practitioner, so that you can obtain personalized treatment for your case. Most of the natural therapies can be safely employed at the same time, however, it is highly recommended that you consult your physician first. Some **herbal treatments may inhibit the oral contraceptives** as well as certain medication.

The author of this book does not claim that reading this book alone will make you lose weight. However, it does offer an overview of alternative and natural remedies that you may find very helpful.

Ensure that all of the natural food supplements that you purchase are natural and organic. It is highly recommended to research the brand first. Read the instructions provided, **and be mindful** of the doses recommended, and if you have any doubts about the intake, consult a specialist who will design individual treatment according to your case.

Even though this book already mentions the **general precautions** listed with each remedy, make sure that your condition allows you to safely use those remedies, and always double-check with the instructions provided with each remedy or natural supplement that you choose to buy and use.

Chapter 1 Natural Weight Control

Phytotherapy (=herbalism) is now the "thing" in the alternative medicine field. This is a practice that combines traditional and scientific methods to provide safer, cheaper, and more effective treatments to health conditions and aid in optimal body nourishment that ultimately leads to a longer, better life. For centuries, plant-based substances and extracts have been utilized for medical reasons. However, it was not until the start of the new millennium that herbs, fruits, vegetables, and trees were deeply studied for the purpose of identifying scientifically backed natural alternatives for treatments, and surprisingly, weight loss. Now, thanks to the buzz that the Paleo diet is creating, it seems that the old, good phytotherapy is back as well!

I always highly recommend phytotherapy for natural weight control and management. You can also use it to improve your skin condition, stimulate your metabolism, and restore your energy levels. If you would like to quit or to reduce coffee and caffeine drinks and are tired of endless resources recommending only green tea(yes, we all know that green tea can help us burn fat!) you will never get bored with herbal infusions that phytotherapy can offer. Not only has it been proven to be effective and safe, it is a healthier alternative. Anybody can try it; it comes in capsules, tablets, juices extracts, tincture, and patented infusions – all as natural dietary supplements. Phytotherapy basically follows the intense use of phytochemicals, or phytonutrients, found in plants. These are the powerful antioxidants that have been found to be a natural enemy of weight accumulation. Through the use of these natural substances, fat elimination and release are induced, calorie conversion minimized, *crazy* appetite appeased, plus energy and muscle development are enhanced.

Phytotherapy is alkaline. It can be a great addition to any alkaline diet program.

In this chapter, I list the most effective natural weight loss remedies that you can try, complete with their most pronounce benefits. I have also included slight setbacks that you may encounter, so that you can take precautionary measures, something that I can never stress enough. Also, please do remember that if you are taking any kind of medication (standard, medical treatments), or even if you are doing a similar, natural treatment (e.g. homeopathy) you should always consult your doctor first. Some herbal treatments may interfere with standard prescription drugs as well as with natural treatments (it can happen when overdosed as well). Too much of a good thing can also become a bad thing, so please, be careful—it's your body.

Artichoke Extract Tablets

Artichokes are good for low-calorie diets; however, when processed into an artichoke extract tablet, it becomes an even more powerful remedy for weight control and management. The tablet is made from the extracted leaves and is typically recommended as a remedy for gastrointestinal problems, such as health conditions concerning the kidney, liver, and digestive track.

As a natural weight loss supplement, it is effective in controlling cholesterol absorption. This is done by inducing bile secretion that can minimize cholesterol distribution to the organs and blood stream. High amounts of cholesterol in the body are one of the primary risk factors for genetic obesity. Also, it is associated with metabolic inefficiency, which means fewer calories are burned.

So, even if you don't like artichokes (personally, I love them, but I know people who hate them!), you can still incorporate them into your diet as a powder, tablets, or capsules. You will also do your liver a big favor and if you want to restore your energy levels naturally, artichoke extract is great. According to Traditional Chinese Medicine, a healthy liver means balanced emotions and no anger. This organ is also related to healthy eyesight. As a kid, I used to suffer from uveitis attacks, and naturopathic doctors who actually saved my eyesight, also worked with phytotherapy concoctions, and artichoke extract was one of the ingredients to help cleanse my liver (I had been given way too many antibiotics as a kid; it wasn't because of alcohol!).

Now, back to weight loss: artichoke powder is a natural, green, and super alkaline supplement that you can add to your juices, salads, and smoothies. You can also use artichoke tablets and capsules (first, research the brand). It can be a great solution if you are busy or travelling.

I need to warn you that artichoke extract tablets are NOT recommended for pregnant women and children under twelve years old. People allergic to daisies and marigolds should consult their doctor first, to rule out possible adverse reactions.

Pineapple Extract Tablets

Many people are not even aware that such supplements exist. Pineapple extract, more commonly known as bromelain, is mainly sourced from the stem of the plant. It has been used for a wide range of conditions, from mild nasal and skin inflammations to several dreaded diseases, such as cancer and pulmonary edema.

Pineapple extract is also recommended for anti-cellulite and fat-burning treatments, as it successfully stimulates both. As a weight loss remedy, bromelain works by speeding up digestion for quicker fat splitting, elimination, and cholesterol flushing. Energy release from the cellular level has also been observed in some studies. If you have a present digestive problem, I urge you to consult your doctor first, as its fiber content might be too much for your body to handle, which can lead to dehydration and diarrhea.

I have personally used pineapple extract capsules in my *burn cellulite* efforts, and it worked great for me. It's not that I don't like eating pineapple, but there are dozens of other fruits and vegetables that I prefer, this is why I always end up skipping it. Getting pineapple powder capsules was an excellent idea, and I still use it occasionally.

Camelina

Camelina, or Camelina Sativa, is traditionally cultivated as a source of cooking essential oils. Many European countries also consider it a major animal feed. Camelina Oil can be considered a natural anti-aging remedy, as its seeds are actually one of the richest sources of Omega-3 fatty acid and also a decent source for natural vitamin E. If you want to improve your memory, nourish your brain, or do better with your exams, I urge you to try camilina oil!

As a weight loss remedy, camelina fights cholesterol build-up, especially in the liver and heart, essential in restoring the body's efficiency in fat elimination. In addition, it also enhances metabolism to consume more calories. Don't use it if you are

15

caffeine-sensitive. Camelina is actually similar to green tea, it is a natural, soft stimulant and is also recommended in fat-burning treatments.

Citrus aurantium

Citrus aurantium, more popularly known as bitter orange, is a common adjuvant ingredient of many weight loss supplements due to its potent fat-burning properties. Before it was used for weight loss, it's been a widely cultivated fruit for essential oil and perfume-making. As a weight loss remedy, it increases the metabolic function through thermogenesis, a process where the body produces a higher temperature to burn more calories at a shorter period. Fat breakdown on a cellular level is also more efficient, yet my opinion is that the best benefit for obese people is its effective appetite suppressing properties.

It is worth noting that people with a sensitive stomach may feel slight discomfort until they get used to taking the supplement. Increased blood pressure and heart rate can also occur. Please, consult your physician before you start using this supplement.

None of the above-mentioned possible side effects are considered 'chronic', however, it is still highly recommended that safety precautions are followed when using natural supplements; the fact that they are natural does not mean that one can abuse them. Many phytotherapists I know recommend using Citrus aurantium for a limited period of time (for example for 3-4 weeks), when a person is undergoing a weight loss diet or program. However, it should never be abused, or consumed without consulting a specialist. Citrus aurantium certainly does sound tempting as one of its main properties includes burning more calories.

Fasolina

Fasolina is virtually unknown as it is usually referred to by its common and scientific names, white kidney bean extract and *Phaseoulus vulgaris*, respectively. It also refers to common beans, such as string beans and garden beans. As an alternative medicine, it is usually used as a natural diuretic.

As a weight loss remedy, fasolina blocks fat to prevent absorption into the body through insulin regulation. Many athletic organizations also include this supplement to their nutrition programs as an energy stabilizer.

There are certain possible unwanted reactions that overdosing of fasolina may cause, and these include nausea and diarrhea. It is important to ensure precise measurements when using these treatments, personally recommended by a specialist according to your medical history. Fasolina is also recommended after weight loss regimes as it can help maintain your ideal weight, so that you don't get absorbed by the vicious circle of putting the weight back on.

Fucus

Fucus, or Fucus vesiculosus, is an aquatic algae abundant in the Mediterranean Sea and other parts of the world, mostly the zones of rocky seashores. Also called kelp and bladderwrack, it contains powerful antioxidants in the form of fucoidan.
Fucus improves digestion and balances cholesterol levels in the heart and blood. I also highly recommend this for people who undergo active training programs, as it relieves muscle pains caused by excessive stretching and pulling. Fucus is rich in vitamins: C, B1, B2, B6 and B12, and can even prevent muscle cramps.

Be careful, and don't pick the wrong brand that contains higher amounts of heavy metals, like mercury. Many manufacturers use additives to preserve the potency in every bottle. Be extra cautious if you are pregnant, breastfeeding, or have recently undergone surgery. You can use fucus as an herbal infusion or take focus tablets or capsules; personally, I prefer the second option as I don't like the taste of fucus tea.

Garcinia Cambogia Extract

Garcinia Cambogia extract is the current diet craze, because of its really promising weight loss benefit, especially those bordering obesity. In fact, I suggest that you try this first, as it will be a great help to fight the so-called 'binge-eating' impulses.

Garcinia Cambogia suppresses appetite by releasing neurons that control hunger and cravings. Garcinia has one outstanding component that also converts more fats for energy consumption while blocking most of fat intakes. You may find it amazing that this extract possesses all features of an excellent weight loss supplement that you are perhaps looking for: In fact, it could be called 'all in one extract'!

This extract is not recommended for pregnant or nursing women, or people with signs of Alzheimer's disease, as the condition might worsen as seen on some clinical studies.

Mate Extract

Mate, or yerba mate, is a powerful stimulant used to relieve mental and physical exhaustion brought about by heavy workouts and excessive training. I consider this a really good way to pump up the blood to generate more energy and enhance the muscles' efficiency in burning calories, primarily due to its high caffeine level.

Mate's benefit as an appetite suppressant, is amplified when processed in the form of a liquid supplement and tonic. This is in addition to its rich antioxidant content.

Not much is known about its side effects, but on my assessment, some minor digestive problems might occur on long-term usage and if you don't really tolerate caffeine drinks, then abstain from using mate, as it may make you too nervous.

Yerba Mate (or *Hierba Mate* in Spanish) is a traditional drink and a very important social ritual in countries like Argentina, Uruguay, and Bolivia. It is normally consumed via *bombilla* or as Argentinians pronounce it, *bombisha*, which at first glance looks a bit like a pipe. Yerba Mate is also sold in tea bags and consumed just like normal tea. Many Argentineans, including one of my best friends who introduced me to mate, would object to it, though as it would go against their well-established, 'cultural mate' rituals of drinking mate via 'una bombisha'.

Its taste is very bitter, it's a bit similar to green tea, and not everyone enjoys it unless they're used to it. This is why mate extract capsules may be a preferred more of usage for some people—capsules or tablets are also less time-consuming.

Choose your preferred way of using mate, but if you happen to have any Argentinean or Uruguayan natives around—ask them to teach you how to prepare yerba mate in a proper way. And remember, do not overdose! Argentineans are used to drinking mate, but you may find it too strong! If you overdo mate, the effects will be the same as after overdoing coffee. You may get too shaky and too nervous. Brrr...

Orthosiphon Aristatus

Orthosiphon Aristatus is a really powerful antioxidant. Many consumers are more familiar with this Southeast Asian herb as Cat's Whiskers. It has been a popular remedy for diabetes and kidney stone treatment in the East, but in Europe and in the U.S., it is starting to build its reputation as an effective weight loss supplement.

Its potential benefit against cellulite is definitely something to watch out for and it is a great 2 in 1 remedy: anti-cellulite as well as weight loss stimulating. It works as a natural lymphatic drainage and can be a great remedy for someone suffering from slow venous circulation, water retention, or even inflammation.

This is generally safe, but if you have ever had allergies to other plants, you should take it fulltime only after monitoring for adverse reactions. Even though there is no study to confirm that Orthosiphon can be dangerous during pregnancy, many naturopathic doctors recommend abstaining from using it while pregnant. <u>Prolonged intake, just like in case of most of the remedies mentioned in this book, is never recommended</u>.

Papaya Extract

Papaya is renowned for its high dietary fiber content that promotes healthy digestion and lower cholesterol. As a weight loss remedy, you can also use its extracted form.

Papaya extract helps in reducing fat absorption from digested foods, which means less fat will be stored in the body. It also helps in flushing out caloric components from other sources.

There are many other benefits of using Papaya Extract: healthier-looking, beautiful skin, improved digestion, increased energy levels, reduced inflammation, and stronger hair.

Remember that eating papaya fruits is not the same as using papaya extract. As for the latter, there are certain contraindications, e.g. pregnancy, thrombosis, and hemophilia. It may also interfere with anticoagulants. Make sure that using papaya extract is 100% safe in your case! If it's not—abstain from using it.

If you are prone to allergies, here comes another precaution to bear in mind: papaya extract may provoke occasional rashes and swellings. Again, it all depends on a person; everyone is different.

Meadowsweet (*Spirae ulmaria L.)*

Meadowsweet, or also commonly known as mead wort, has long been cultivated for its salicylic acid content, a substance that is widely used as a natural replacement for pain killers, such as aspirin, diuretics, and analgesics. Until now, many people still use it to treat peptic ulcers and bladder infections.

For those of you who want to lose weight, meadowsweet acts as an enhancer of the digestive system, which reduces fat absorption and minimizes cholesterol intake. If you are currently under a strenuous fitness program, perhaps you could try this out, as it will soothe aching muscles and strengthen your respiratory system.

If you are looking for natural anti-cellulite treatments or are suffering from water retention, this herb can really increase your quality of life!
Meadowsweet is also a really powerful antioxidant and can form part of your natural cleanse program. Personally, I know many

natural beauty therapists who recommend this herb to rejuvenate the skin and to grow strong and healthy hair.

There are certain precautions and interactions: asthma (should be used with caution), and it may interfere with standard anti-inflammatory drugs as well as anticoagulant drugs.

Shan Zha

Shan Zha, often called *hawthorn berry* in the U.S., comes in many supplement forms, most common in 160 to 1,000 milligram capsules. I think it is a bit hyped up as a weight loss supplement only without taking away from its actual benefits. Many brands market it as a fat burner, but the truth is that it is not.

As a weight loss remedy, hawthorn berry reduces weight by eliminating the body's excess sodium. As a result of the sodium being expelled, your water retention also lowers, and the fluid that makes you look bloated and rotund is flushed out. It is also great for anti-cellulite treatments and helps treat water retention.

Shan Za is also a natural remedy used in anxiety treatments and is also recommended for people undergoing nervousness because of stopping smoking. As it is caffeine-free, with some great relaxing properties, it is a great 2 in 1 remedy for those who wish to stimulate weight-loss as well as prevent anxiety. In fact, not everyone can use supplements like mate, guarana, or cola: Some people just experience the whole collection of effects, similar to those when overdosing on coffee or alcohol: Shaking, sweating, increased heart beat, and even panic attacks. If you know that you are one of those sensitive individuals who can easily experience some unpleasant reactions as mentioned above, then shan za will be a great alternative for you. It is very important to know which type you are and select your natural remedy carefully.

Mild headache, nausea, and occasional erroneous heart beats might happen, but only when this weight loss supplement is taken in the wrong dosage. Stick to not more than 1,800 milligrams (better if you double-check with your physician), especially when you do not have excessive water retention to begin with.

Now, it's time to analyze your situation, and select your preferred remedy and test it. As I have already mentioned there are many 2 in 1 remedies that will bring more health benefits that you can imagine. Trust me, having your little natural remedy friend will make you more prepared and determined to stick to your healthy lifestyle and exercise program: Physically, you will feel better and less food craving temptations will occur, you will also feel stronger mentally and emotionally. If you have such a powerful natural remedy on your side, what can possibly go wrong? The only thing to remember is to take it regularly, as recommended in the instructions, but for someone as determined like you, my reader and friend, it shouldn't be a problem.

And again, please remember that reading this book alone can't substitute a consultation that you should have with your physician before employing any of the phytotherapy supplements mentioned in this chapter. This is what I always do myself (I ask my doctor, yes!). Also, obtaining a personalized treatment is not something that you can get from a book or an article, still, it can work as a great introduction.

Chapter 2 Increase Your Energy Levels

Why is it important for someone on a battle against weight increase to maintain high energy levels? First, with all the strenuous physical activities that you will deal with along the way, perhaps lasting for months, you are far away from succeeding if all that you now feel is laziness and fatigue. It is inevitable for many people to feel weakness, mental fatigue, and reduced focus during the first few weeks, due to the quick expulsion of fat deposits and water from the body, new ways of eating and such a major shift in training regime. Trust me, I have been there myself. You cannot expect to continue your workouts when feeling like a blanched vegetable.

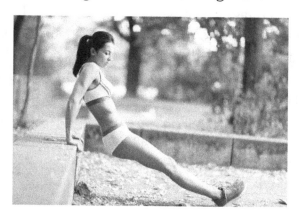

Second, nutrition deficiency is a common setback of a major diet shift. You need to revitalize your cellular energy from the core, by filling up with fuel in the form of five scientifically proven natural energy toners. Lastly, increasing your energy means increasing your biological capacity to burn calories. This is especially true for those muscles that will do the work, while you train and while you sleep.

Here are five food supplements that I highly recommend for weight loss and weight control. They will keep you nicely energized, so that you will be successful in your exercise programs and won't be tempted to stuff yourself with unhealthy foods: *My body is asking me to feed it with chocolate, waffles, biscuits, ice-cream, and other enemies...* In fact, this feeling will be banned when you prepare yourself accordingly with some super powerful and natural energy boosters.

Guarana

Guarana is native to South America, and it produces seeds that contain a high concentration of caffeine, making it a more effective stimulant and muscle relaxant than coffee. As a matter of fact, guarana's seeds have twice the caffeine level of coffee beans.

On initial scientific assessments, its antioxidant is considered supreme, which makes it a candidate for the top superfood ever discovered. Many new energy drinks now use guarana as their primary source of caffeine, although, if you really want to get the full benefit of its antioxidant, I suggest using the supplement form. Guarana also brings mental stimulation and is also recommended for cases of intellectual work, exams, excessive studying, etc. Make sure you always have some spare guarana tablets in your gym bag, and use it before workouts so as to increase fat burning. It will definitely make your workout more efficient and take the best of you; you will be surprised at your success.

It is considered as generally safe, although, some clinical observations have included lowered platelets as its side effects. If you are caffeine-sensitive, you shouldn't take guarana as it will over stimulate you increasing your heartbeat. From my own experience: I can't take guarana, it just makes me too nervous. I only use it very occasionally (for example with my smoothies).

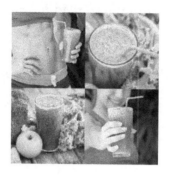

Spiruline

Spiruline, or more commonly known as *spirulina*, is a powerful cyanobacterium with impressive levels of antioxidants. It is usually sold in powder and tablet forms, and either one works perfectly in releasing cellular energy.

You can use the dried form as a replacement to protein shakes as it contains up to 70% complete protein (meaning, it has the complete spectrum of amino acids vital to muscle growth).

Unlike guarana, spiruline is not a stimulant and is caffeine free. It's one of those safe food supplements, famous for its high nourishing effects, and many naturopathic doctors recommend it as a regular food supplement. I like to use it with my smoothies.

Taking spiruline means making sure that your body gets all the nutrients it needs; it will help bring balance and revitalize naturally. If taken before a meal, spiruline will help suppress excessive hunger and burn fat.

Spiruline will also help detoxify your body from excessive unhealthy foods, environmental pollution, and other unhealthy indulging. It will also stimulate your immune system and make you stronger. If you are vegetarian, spiruline should not be omitted in your diet as it is a natural source of protein and iron.

Be sure that you pick a credible brand, so that there are no toxicity issues. Enjoy your superfood!

Royal Jelly

For sure, you are familiar with royal jelly as more and more food supplements now add this to their labels to aid in energy restoration. I think every man or woman who undergoes strenuous workouts should include it on her nutritional program.

Royal jelly is the secretion of honey bees, meant to serve as the ultimate source of nutrition of their queen and larvae. For humans, its high B vitamin levels and amino acids work as really promising muscle enhancers and anti-aging agents. What made it a real household name is its aphrodisiac and memory enhancing effects. It is also used to prevent colds and flu.

Some people may experience an allergic reaction when using Royal Jelly. Luckily, I never got any of those. I must say that my overall experience with Royal jelly was good, and I would also recommend it to you if you want to strengthen your immune system or if you are prone to colds and flu.

Kola

The name should give you a clue. It belongs to the evergreen species abundant in tropical countries. Its seeds are very rich in caffeine, making it an excellent physical and mental stimulant to keep you pumping day in and day out. You should have realized by now that this was originally an essential ingredient in making carbonated drinks—cola to be exact.

It inhibits fatigue and hunger, which also makes this supplement one of my favorite natural energy enhancers and muscle stimulant. Some people suffer "Seasonal Effective Disorder" i.e. lack of energy and motivation, during winter, or

in particularly cold Far Northern countries, and are more pı
to staying in, overeating and exercise procrastination.

If you are not used to other sources of caffeine, it might m
you feel nauseous at the first few weeks. Your condition ı
stabilize after some time, but if you are caffeine sensitive
can't take caffeine for any other reason (e.g. pregnancy
hypertension), abstain from using kola and choose spiruline
royal jelly instead.

From my own experience: I can't take Kola, just like I can't tɛ
guarana really. They make me way too nervous. But I kn
people who benefit a lot from using Kola, so I guess tl
depending on which category you fall into, you may choose yc
remedy.

Ginseng

Many experts might disagree with me, but I consider ginseng overrated, despite its proven potency as a natural energy enhancer. It is overrated not because it delivers less than what many people claim, but because many herbs made into supplements will deliver the same benefits anyway.

Nonetheless, the ginseng root is a very rich source of a substance used as a stimulant both on a physical and a mental level. The treatment of ginseng should not exceed a month and is normally done once or twice a year (at the most) to stimulate the body's vital force.

Many naturopathic specialists claim that the best time of the year to use ginseng is in the springtime or fall when the body needs more energy to get used to the change of temperatures. Of course, it also depends on the individual needs—everyone knows when their body needs the overall revitalization, and ginseng is great for that as it is rich in amino acids, vitamin C, and vitamin B. It is also known as a very potential aphrodisiac. There are different kinds of ginseng, and it's of paramount importance to research the brand to make sure that only a good quality, natural ginseng supplement is taken.

Nausea and mild headaches might occur for people with sensitivity to certain substances, but that is rare. However, some people feel over stimulated when taking ginseng, and generally it is not recommended for people prone to anxiety, insomnia, or nervousness. Some Macrobiotic Diet experts say that ginseng is definitely not a female stimulant as many females may react with: headaches and increased nervousness. This is what happened to me, and I can tell you that it's not my stimulant. But again, it seems to work well for many people, and I even know doctors who recommend ginseng treatment once a year.

Chapter 3 Teas for Weight Loss

Teas are widely used alternatives for unhealthy chemical slimming pills because they deliver faster results and give fewer side effects. It is very important to use those teas regularly as an addition to a balanced diet and variegated exercise plan. Some people mistakenly believe that quantity is what matters, and then, tend to overdo the weight loss teas. The common complaints in taking weight loss teas in exaggerated amounts are: nausea, diarrhea, and even headaches, and so even though these are 'only teas', precautions should be taken.

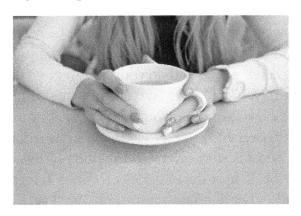

In my opinion, moderation is always the key; some teas may stimulate weight loss but should not be considered the ultimate solution; one will be more successful in the long run if determined to a weight loss plan. Combining different kinds of weapons in a regular way will definitely help and natural weight loss teas are a nice addition that will further help lose unwanted pounds.

Try out my top tips and drink your way through to a slimmer body.

Green Tea

I am sure you have heard of this one, so I will keep it brief. Green tea is highly favored in the natural weight loss industry because of its very potent thermogenesis properties. Its catechin called EGCG, which makes it a powerful cancer prevention as well, is touted to be a strong fat burner that increases internal temperature, which in effect, enhances metabolism.

Just by drinking a cup of green tea every day, you are already stimulating your metabolism and treating your body with some very powerful antioxidants.

Green tea, as well as red tea, is considered to be a natural fat burner. If you manage to replace at least one daily cup of coffee with some green tea, you will do your body a great favor, and in the long run, you will also be more energized. Green tea contains some levels of theine but won't over stimulate as much as coffee. Whereas coffee can give you an immediate boost of energy, this boost is very soon accompanied by a sudden fall of energy, and this is how dependency on coffee is created. Green tea, on the other hand, offers a more subtle physical and mental stimulation that lasts longer and is not accompanied by an abrupt fall of energy.

Peppermint Tea

This tea is an excellent support when fighting strong urge to eat. As an appetite suppressant, it eliminates harmful cravings that can throw your diet off-track. If you have an inefficient digestion, this will also help tremendously in expelling excess water and fat deposits. Mint tea can be a great addition to green tea as well: you will obtain an antioxidant and naturally revitalizing drink that is traditionally called the Moroccan tea.

Avoid sugar though, it may be tempting to make your green and mint tea super sweet just like the Moroccans do, but you need to watch out for that. You want to lose weight! Moreover, if you add some mint herbs or a mint tea bag to green tea, you will change its bitter favor into a nice, minty one, and so, it will be easier to combat the temptation of using sugar.

Oolong Tea

Oolong is a type of mushroom that is traditionally used to treat different medical conditions such as osteoporosis, heart disease, and tooth decay. As a weight loss tea, it reduces the cholesterol level in the blood, stimulates metabolism, and it also makes fat consumption by the muscles faster and more efficient. Oolong tea contains caffeine, so it stimulates the central nervous system. If you are nervous by nature or caffeine intolerant, then avoid oolong tea or take it only in moderate amounts.

Star Anise Tea (The Chinese Star Anise Species)

This is not my palate's most preferred tea, but as it is a very effective remedy for weight loss efforts, I definitely recommend this. It enhances digestion, which makes expulsion of fats and water easier. If you are having a problem eliminating water retention, this tea is for you as it also stimulates the sluggish lymphatic system. It also stimulates elimination of toxins, so you will regain your energy levels naturally.

Make sure that you research the brand, and pick up the Chinese Star Anise, as the Japanese is toxic and detrimental to health and shouldn't be consumed.

Many phytotherapists also use star anise to treat flu, rheumatism, and inflammation. It is also widely used in Indian, Chinese, and Vietnamese cuisine. Personally, what I find fascinating about all the natural remedies is that they are extremely multifunctional and that there is always something new to be discovered about them. I also have lots of respect for phytotherapists, commonly called herbalists, as it is really a life-long study.

Rose Tea

It does more than just relax the mind with its wonderful aroma; it also relaxes the muscles to keep them prepared for another day's fight. It has all the potent vitamins–A, B3, C, D, and E. When combined with green tea or oolong tea, it can be an even more powerful weight loss tea.

Moreover, it cleanses the liver and gall bladder, promoting bile flow. It is considered to be a great antioxidant remedy, and it is widely used in Ayurvedic medicine. If you also suffer from fluid retention and experience overall tiredness, you should definitely try rose tea on a regular basis.

Its calming properties make it a perfect choice for insomnia, stress, or anxiety victims. I personally find its flavor and fragrance extremely relaxing. Add to it its therapeutic properties, and you have a great, multifunctional remedy!

Experiment with different teas, so as to be sure that you create a variety in your weight loss efforts. Teas can be also consumed cold—you can treat yourself to a natural and healthy delicious energy drink.

You can also use teas for smoothies: e.g. green tea, mint tea, or rose tea when cooled down can be a great base for smoothies, who said that it has to be milk? Have you ever tried green tea + strawberries + cherries + pineapple + banana smoothie? It is a really powerful weight loss stimulant and is also great for cellulite and sluggish circulation.

Interested in juices and smoothies? Read on through the next chapter!

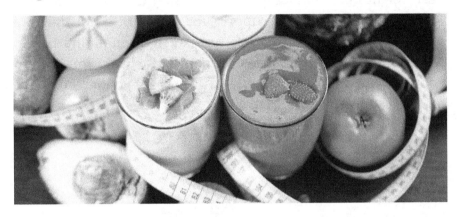

Chapter 4 Juices for Weight Loss

The idea of juicing fruits, vegetables, and herbs to lose weight and maintain a desirable one revolves around the principles of detoxification and meal replacement. Weight loss juices are the best weight maintenance essentials as they do not only possess fat burning and appetite suppressing properties, but they are also rich in nutrients that are needed in maintaining health while all the physical changes happen. But why do you need to support your weight loss battle with juices if you already have all these supplements and teas?

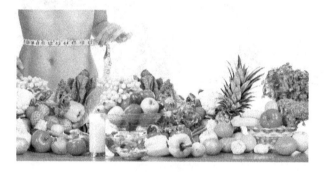

First, juices, as well as smoothies, are heavy meal replacements that you certainly need to take to keep something in your tummy while at the same time, eating less unhealthy, processed foods. You have to eat, but eat wisely. The ultimate way to do that is to eat, or for this matter, drink liquid meals. If you include vegetable juices on a daily basis, you will drastically remove the danger of possible food cravings, and you will be also full of energy as well as preventing many serious diseases.

Second, juices are very effective detoxifiers to eliminate all the accumulated toxins in your body. With green smoothies especially, you will feel younger and will certainly look younger. But what does detoxification have to do with weight loss?

The fat cannot burn calories efficiently and convert them into energy sources if the liver, together with digestive organs, are full of toxins. You need to restore their optimum function to revitalize your optimum metabolism.

Lastly, you can get the natural weight loss properties of herbs, fruits, and vegetables by extracting them, and what else is the best way to do that but by juicing?

The list of possible juice and smoothie variations is just endless, and your imagination is the only limit of what you can do.
To begin with, if your main objective is weight loss and rejuvenation, take the following tips into consideration when creating your juices and smoothies:

-Use only organic fruits and vegetables; you want to revitalize, and so, you don't want any chemicals or artificial food preservatives in your juices;

- Avoid procrastination: juicing or making smoothies may seem to be a bit time-consuming when you first start, but the long-term benefits that you get will actually be extremely rewarding: you will avoid many conditions like low energy levels, and in the long-run, even possible doctor appointments. Each time, when you make a juice, tell yourself that you are investing time in your health and that you want to be brimming with energy and vitality even when you are eighty! Life is so beautiful that not a single day should be lost! You will be also saving money: regular juicing will be the best beauty treatment that you can ultimately get—and all this naturally, from the inside;

-Make sure you pick up a juicer and a blender that you are comfortable with using, after all, you two will be spending quite a lot of time together. Finding the right blender is as important as finding a car that works properly. You also may consider investing in a good quality juicer or blender that will 'last forever' no matter how much you juice and that is also easy to clean.

- If you know you hate preparing juices, just buy them. How many times have you had a drink or a coffee out? With so many places that offer fresh juices and smoothies, if you cannot make yourself one at home, at least make sure you grab one on the way to work.

What to juice/blend?

An experienced 'juicing guru' would say that you can juice pretty much everything.

To begin with, if you want to achieve balance, health, and weight loss, choose fruits and vegetables that are highly alkalizing that is low in sugar and high in minerals—these include:

Juicing Ingredients:

1. Alkaline vegetables: carrot, cucumber, garlic, onion, pepper, green spinach, broccoli, and sea veggies. When juicing, try to focus on vegetables as much as possible, especially leafy greens.

   You can learn more on juicing for my other book: "Alkaline Juicing" (available on Amazon).

2. Alkaline fruits: grapefruit, lemon, lime, tomato and pomegranates are the best options for juices. Why? Because they are naturally low in sugar and super high in minerals which makes them highly alkalizing fruits, even though their taste is acidic (yes, lemons are alkaline, even though they taste acidic). If you have never heard of the alkaline diet before (it sounds a bit complicated and even faddish at first, but trust me, it's a really common-sense, healthy and balanced lifestyle and it's one of my favorite "Wellness Tools" to work with), go ahead and sign up for your free gifts (it includes easy, printable charts):

www.HolisticWellnessProject.com/alkaline

Blending/Smoothie Ingredients:

Other fruits (here I refer to fruits that are not low in sugar, for example bananas, kiwis) is OK, but don't juice them, but blend them. Use them to create colorful, tasty smoothies. Still, if your goal is weight loss, I would focus 80% on juicing vegetables (or using them in smoothies) or fruit low in sugar and 20% on other fruits- I would use them as a natural, healthy treat (kiwis, bananas, pineapples etc.)

More suggestions:

-If you like smoothies experiment with coconut milk, coconut water, rice milk, oat milk, and almond milk (super alkaline!);

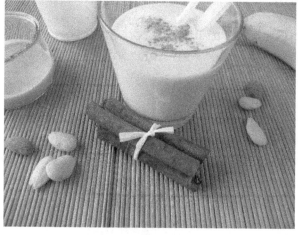

-Soya lecithin granules, alfalfa powder, as well as barley grass can be a nice addition to a juice or a smoothie and increase its nutritional value.

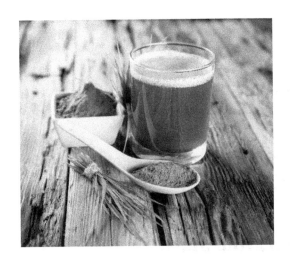

Check out some of my favorite juices:

Green Smoothie Smash It Morning Energy

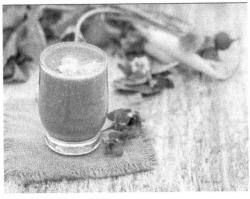

This is a great breakfast recipe, and with high iron and magnesium levels you can be certain that you will keep your energy levels high and will successfully do your morning workout:

Blend:

- 1 cup almond milk
- ½ cup spinach leaves
- 1 banana
- ½ avocado
- + add one teaspoon of alfalfa powder + (optional) juice of 1 lime or lemon

Beautiful Body and Mind Juice

If drunk regularly, not only will it help to stimulate weight loss, but it will also improve your skin condition giving it a healthy, tanned-like look. High levels of vitamin C and ginger will help you prevent colds and flu:

Place the following ingredients through the juicer (preferably low speed juicer):

- 2 carrots
- 1 apple
- 1 cup kale
- 1 inch ginger
- 1 grapefruit

Enjoy!

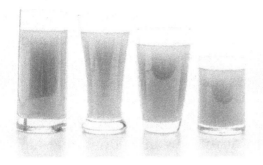

Alkaline Power Green Juice

If you feel low in energy or have indulged in unhealthy choices, take care of your body the way it deserves and give it a nice mix of vitamins and minerals:
Place the following ingredients through the juicer:

- 1 cucumber
- 2 carrots
- 1 zucchini
- 1 cup spinach + add a few drops of fresh lemon juice and (optional) alkaline powder (e.g. alfalfa or barley grass or wheat grass powder)

If you are not a big fan of vegetable juices, try my favorite vegetable cream soup:

Broccoli and Carrot Antioxidant Soup

Use one broccoli and a few carrots (feel free to change the proportions according to your preferences) as well as a little bit of garlic and onion to spice up.

Wash the veggies and cut them into small pieces and put them to boil. Make sure you keep the temperature low, and turn the cooker off when the water starts boiling: You don't want the vegetables to lose their nutrients. Let it cool down a bit, and add some cold-pressed organic olive oil and a few tablespoon of soy milk and any kinds of spices you like (e.g. rosemary).

Blend all the ingredients and enjoy your warm, creamy veggie soup that will be easy to digest, low in calories, and high in nutrients!

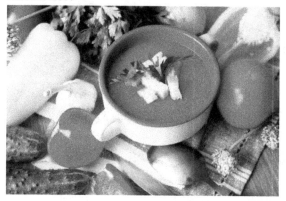

Anti-Cellulite Smoothie

As I have mentioned before, pineapples have some really strong anti-cellulite properties. If apart from unwanted pounds, cellulite is also your enemy, treat yourself to a regular anti-cellulite smoothie:

Blend: one cup of cooled green tea + half cup of almond or rice milk + blueberries+ pineapple (you may choose equal proportions or let one of the fruits dominate).

Creating your own recipes is the fun part though, make sure that you get in habits for shopping for fresh organic fruits and vegetables and get in the habit of making fresh juices. Losing weight in a healthy way and restoring your energy levels will only be a couple of hundreds of long-term benefits that juicing will bring.

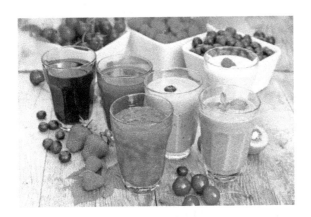

Juices + smoothies are the essence of life; embrace it and enjoy it!

Remember that when preparing a juice, you make the best time investment ever.

Your health will be so grateful that it will pay you with high energy levels and a zest for life! Additional mental benefits that can't be overlooked are: increased creativity and focused mind. It's not only about weight loss.

If you are interested in learning more about smoothies and juices, check out my other books (available in kindle and paperback):

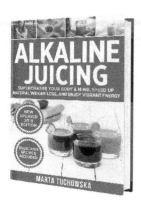

You will find them at:
www.amazon.com/author/mtuchowska
or: www.holisticwellnessproject.com

To sum up, these are the best fruits for weight loss as they are natural low in sugar. Use them in your juices and smoothies. You may even blend them with herbal teas.

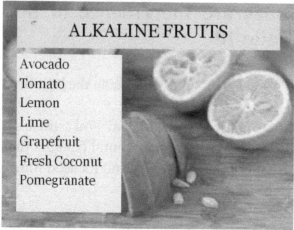

ALKALINE FRUITS

Avocado
Tomato
Lemon
Lime
Grapefruit
Fresh Coconut
Pomegranate

These are great natural supplements that you can mix with your smoothies or salads. If you are pressed for time, just mix them with some clean, filtered water. It's always good to detox!

ALKALINE GRASSES

Wheatgrass
Barley Grass
Kamut Grass
Dog Grass
Shave Grass
Oat Grass

BONUS CHAPTER

Aside from phytotherapy, there are other holistic therapies that you can use to stimulate massive weight loss. This chapter is a free preview of my book: "Essential Oils for Natural Weight Loss". Aromatherapy is one of my favorite natural therapies and I use it every day. It's a great form of holistic self-care that everyone can learn and apply at home. In my book, I share my experiences and show you how to employ aromatherapy for weight loss as well as other imbalances. I focus on emotional eating, something that I used to be a victim of. I offer practical solutions for modern people in the 21st century. People like me and you.

Now, I am not a preacher or guru. I am not telling you what to do. I am telling you what I do. I give you information and inspiration so that you can get started on creating! "Creating what?"-you may ask.

Creating Wellness and making it exciting and fun! Finally, becoming a role model for your family and friends. Let's dive into it.

Essential Oils for your Holistic, Naturopathy Weight Loss Spa

The key to success with aromatherapy treatments is <u>consistency</u>. You should aim to make your own, personalized rituals <u>a part of your lifestyle</u>. There is no need to purchase and use all the oils. I suggest you pick up 1-3 to begin with. If you are new to aromatherapy and unfamiliar with some of the scents, I recommend you visit your local health store/naturopathy or organic store and ask them for some essential oils testers.

When seeking mental and emotional benefits of the EO(=essential oils), I have realized that the best tip that I had once been given by one of my teachers and I am giving you now, is to follow your intuition. It will guide you and it will naturally make you attracted to some oils that you find healing. Still, in the beginning it is good to read a little bit about properties and get some guidance and instructions. This is what this chapter offers you.

Aromatherapy Blends/rules

The basic rules to keep in mind are the following proportions:

-For 15ml of vegetable oil (equals to one tablespoon) add 5- 7 drops of essential oil.

-For 2ml of vegetable oil, add 1 drop of essential oil.

If you are working on the face, use weaker concentrations, especially if you have sensitive skin:

For 30ml of a vegetable oil (or cream) use 1- 2 drops of essential oil.

It also depends on which essential oil you are using. For example, verbena, which is one of my favorites, can be pretty irritating when applied on the face. I normally use only 1 drop of verbena EO in, for more or less, 10 ml of a vegetable oil. I like using this simple blend for night time facial massages: it nourishes my skin and is great for oily complexions, like mine, and at the same time, it prevents headaches, puts me in a good mood, and makes me sleep like a baby. This is my favorite anti-insomnia oil.

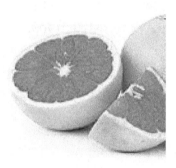

Let's have a look at the army of weight loss essential oils (EO)

GRAPEFRUIT EO (*citrus x paradisi*)

This oil has a whole range of mind and body properties. It works as:

- Antidepressant
- Antiseptic
- Disinfectant
- Diuretic
- Stimulant
- Tonic

Grapefruit EO:

- Energizes you and stimulates your metabolism, and is recommended for periods of fatigue and exhaustion
- Helps curb cravings and prevents binge eating, as well as emotional eating
- Works as a natural anti-cellulite treatment
- Acts as a natural diuretic and prevents water retention
- Works as a natural remedy against food addiction
- Helps eliminate toxins from your body and can also help alleviate hangover
- Stimulates the lymphatic system and venous circulation

I find it to be very uplifting and energizing, and I make sure I use it when mental and emotional stress knocks on my door. I would also recommend it for periods of mental and physical exhaustion- athletes, students, and all active individuals can benefit from using it.

When feeling nervous, I dilute 2-3 drops of grapefruit EO in a tablespoon of VO and apply locally on my solar plexus via a gentle massage.

You can use it topically, as described in the previous chapter, as well as aromatically (inhalation, direct inhalation, or if you do not find it irritating to your skin, you could also apply 1-2 drops on your wrists. This is how I do it as a quick, on the go fix).

An interesting fact about this oil is that on an emotional level, it helps increase self-acceptance and self-confidence and trust in a present moment. Try it; I am sure it will put you in a good mood. The good mood thing can be described in plenty of different ways, as everyone is different and so is their emotional reaction to essential oils really. I just mention the most commonly reported soothing, emotional reactions that most people experience.

IMPORTANT PREUCATION:
- Avoid sunbathing for up to 12 hours after use

LEMON EO (*Citrus limon*)

Here comes another citrus essential oil with plenty of therapeutic properties. Its actions are:

- Anti-anemic
- Antimicrobial
- Antirheumatic
- Antitoxic
- Bactericidal
- Depurative
- Diuretic
- Hypotensive
- Tonic

It acts as a natural diuretic and prevents water retention. It is also great for the immune system and it stimulates white corpuscles.

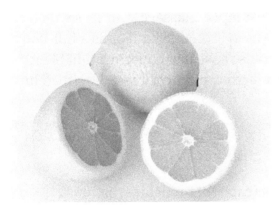

For me, a lemon essential oil fragrance is much better than a cup of coffee, really! I very often use it before my workouts, to enhance motivation (direct inhalation) and after workouts, topically, diluted in sweet almond oil (or any other base oil) as a self-massage treatment after shower.

Do you know this feeling when your brain tells you: "Skip your workout today, you are too tired"? I have noticed that the lemon essential oil usually does the trick for me. I am back on track and all set up for fitness success. Of course, I think it's very important to listen to your body; maybe it really needs some rest? However, in most cases it's just our brain telling us what to do, which normally is couch potato stuff. We don't want to be there, do we? This is why I suggest you confide in this oil for motivation and energy.

I usually include it in my anti-cellulite blends. Very often cellulite is simply a sign of more serious and complex imbalances, such as, for example, slow circulation, water retention, and sluggish lymphatic system (what a delightful combination, eh?).

You can use it locally, for example, massage your legs with a diluted lemon EO, as well as in aromatic bath or as a full-body massage (you may want to use a weaker concentration blend on your face first, or, even better, perform a test described in the previous chapters).

Apart from cellulite, obesity, edema, varicose veins, and slow circulation, this oil is also great for:

- Respiratory system (catarrh, bronchitis, asthma)
- Skin care (acne, greasy skin, insect bites)
- Immune system (flu, colds, infections)

  It can also be used internally (check chapter 6 for more information)

- Avoid sunbathing for up to 12 hours after use

PEPPERMINT EO (*Mentha piperita*)

Here comes another EO that energizes you and stimulates your metabolism. It is great for hot summers as it offers nice, rejuvenating refreshment and fights fatigue that can be provoked by high temperatures.

Personally, I like fragrances obtained by mixing this oil with one of the citrus essential oils (e.g. verbena, lemon, orange, bergamot).

Of course, it's also full of healing properties on its own, as it acts as:

- Anti-inflammatory
- Cephalic (prevents headaches)
- Vasoconstrictor
- Stomachic
- Antiseptic

It is also great for the nervous system, as it soothes migraines, nervous stress, and mental fatigue.

Its refreshing fragrance makes me crave more healthy refreshments! In the summer, I like using this oil after the shower. I normally dilute it in some Aloe Vera gel or organic cream. To finish up the refreshment time, I make myself an energizing smoothie. There is no space for unhealthy food cravings or laziness when this oil takes over!

This oil is pretty powerful and I suggest you use weaker concentrations if you go for a full body massage. 2 drops of this oil can be enough for 1 tablespoon of your chosen vegetable oil. Of course, if you find your blend too weak, you may want to make it stronger. However, wait a few minutes after applying this blend on your body...Mint EO can be too refreshing sometimes! The feeling of coolness can get out of your hands if you overdo this oil for massage.

For a quick fix, use direct inhalation; peppermint essential oil is great for emotional eating prevention.

Preucations:
-Keep away from the eyes, use in small amounts as it may cause irritation of the skin and mucus membranes.

JUNIPER EO (*Juniperus communis*)

If you are looking for natural, detoxifying spa treatments, you have just found your oil! Juniper EO acts as:

- Depurative
- Diuretic
- Tonic

If you want to fight the accumulation of toxins, gout, cellulite, and wish to create your natural weight loss treatments, make sure you include this oil in your blends for regular body massage.

It has a really soft, soothing woody note fragrance, which is a great choice for those of you who are not fond of strong and even overwhelming fragrances.

From my own experience: it offers an immediate relief for a tired body, especially tired and heavy legs. You usually get this feeling if you are in a job that involves either too much sitting in one place (100% sedentary) or standing on your legs for long hours (for example, a hairdresser). I know from my own experience that if you feel that way, you want to get back home, sit down, and probably stuff yourself with FOOD-whatever food there is, as long as it is fast prep...

Since we don't want to take that route, I suggest you resort to juniper essential oil and use it in your blend for body massage after a shower. This is how you will start experiencing its soothing effects on a physical level and will be able to shift your mind towards healthy and nourishing food choices, and maybe even some sports (even though you think you are tired, you can still move your body for 15 minutes and feel great and keep this feeling for the next morning!).

If you decide to use it in inhalations, steam or direct, you will surely notice a positive and uplifting effect on your nervous system, as this oil is great for all stress-related conditions and anxiety.

If you decide to purchase this oil, aside from its weight loss properties you can also use it for:

- Skin and hair care (acne, hair loss, oily complexions)- simply massage your scalp or apply on areas affected (always diluted as mentioned in the previous chapter)

- Immune system: it helps alleviate colds, flu, and other infections; it is a natural anti-inflammatory. In fact, I have used it for chest and throat massage when I was down with the flu and found a relief in it and didn't have to reach for chemical medications (I am not saying that essential oils can substitute standard medications of course, but in this very case, I found juniper oil to be really alleviating). It also helped me relax and sleep better when I was sick.

SWEET ORANGE EO (*Citrus sinensis*)

I can never have enough of citrus oils!

This oil, for sure, forms a part of my lifestyle.

I use it on a regular basis to make sure I stay healthy, vibrant, and slim (again, have you noticed the order of those adjectives? Holistic health will always result in a balanced body!).

As a weight loss essential oil, it stimulates lymphatic and digestive system.

Just a few words on the lymphatic system: it makes sure that toxins are eliminated from, not accumulated in our body. It also must function properly in order to take care of our immune system. The lymphatic system, when not functioning properly, leads to a series of health problems. Some of them might be perceived as a simple beauty defect, for example, cellulite or edema. But the truth is, that these are only the signs of a deeper and more serious problem that should be treated at its root.

The simple steps that you can take to take better care of your lymphatic system, include:

-Healthy and balanced nutrition (I recommend an alkaline diet inspired eating plan)

-Regular exercise (there is no getting away from this one!)

-Getting treated to a lymphatic drainage massage.Commit yourself to a regular massage with diluted essential oils, such as, for example, *Citrus sinesis*, or in plain English: Sweet Orange essential oil.

Aside from its detoxifying properties that act on a physical level, it is also an amazing remedy to soothe your nervous system. As you have surely figured out, either from your own experience, or after reading what I have written so far, the nervous system and the digestive system and, of course, your own, conscious decisions and food choices and even actions you take, are all **INTERCONNECTED**.

This is why I am pretty sure that your nervous system will be more than happy to accommodate Sweet Orange essential oil. It's really great for fighting nervous tension and stress. I also use it to induce better sleep: I use either massage (for example, a quick neck massage to loosen up tension accumulated there) or I just put 1- 2 drops on an old towel (if I put it on the pillow or sheets directly, it may come out as a stain that is really difficult to remove) and put it on my pillow. Sleep like a baby trick! Balance your emotions and mood and choose how you feel!

So, to sum up, you have just met multifunctional oil, that acts as a natural lymphatic drainage, is great for fighting water retention, and can make you feel lighter in your body.

All it takes is to use a few drops of it in your chosen vegetable base oil and massage your body, while inhaling the amazing, soothing fragrance that this oil has. On a mental and emotional level, it fights stress and induces better sleep.

If you decide to purchase this oil, here are other uses:

- Skin care- a natural remedy for oily complexions
- Respiratory system- brings a relief for those suffering from colds, bronchitis, and flu

- Immune system-since it helps stimulate the lymphatic system, if applied regularly, it helps prevent infections and results in overall higher energy levels.

  Precautions: avoid direct sun exposure for up to 10-12 hours

GERANIUM EO (*Pelargonium graveolens*):

I familiarized myself with this oil when doing my basic training in Swedish Massage. One of my teachers was a big fan of this oil. At school, they always had it for sale among other amazing bottles of natural health and beauty products, which quite naturally, I was really attracted to. At that time, I suffered from low energy levels and water retention. I felt like my legs were really, really heavy. This was due to the fact that I broke away from my healthy fitness routine and I kept blaming lack of time and just could not get back on track. I talk about it in my book: *Cellulite Killers*.

Anyway, to cut a long story short, when you feel bad in your body it's hard to take action. My teacher recommended geranium oil, something that she has been using for many years and she told me about a myriad of health and beauty benefits that it offers.

First of all, it forms an important part of natural weight loss treatments, as it has strong energizing and anti-edema properties. It acts as:

- Anti-inflammatory
- Diuretic

61

- Natural lymphatic drainage
- Circulatory system stimulant

If you suffer from cellulite, edema, stretch marks, etc., I strongly suggest you add it to your blends.

Other properties that it possesses are great for the mind and emotions, as it acts as:
- Antidepressant
- Stimulant (adrenal cortex)- it is a natural mood enhancer and helps us feel stronger when confronting everyday problems and stress that life throws at us
- Helps connect with the *here and now* and induces a highly meditative state, where you can communicate with your subconscious mind

Talking about the subconscious mind- it is this part of our mind that collects certain data and information that we may not be aware of is even there, for example: colors, names, people, events, as well as fragrances from the past...!

The reason why I mention this is simple: when experimenting with essential oils, sooner or later, you will come across the oil that takes you back to the past. In my case, it is geranium essential oil. When I was a little girl, I used to vacation over at my grandparents house, and my late grandpa was a big fan of plants. He has quite a few geranium plants on his balcony. Perhaps this is why, geranium oil is one of my favorite oils and it makes me feel really relaxed, secure, and protected!

Conclusion

Thank you again for taking your time and interest in my book! I truly enjoyed writing it, and I hope that it has met your demands. I also hope that it has inspired you to get started on something new! Maintaining an attractive figure and staying within a healthy weight are not only important in making good impressions. It's not only about **how you look** but also about **how you feel**.

Watching your weight and size is essential in ensuring longevity in health and balance. When you start your weight loss program, it is always important to remember that you need to eat balanced meals and have regular exercise. I would also suggest replacing the word *diet* with the word *lifestyle*! Being healthy in a holistic way is not only about losing weight. It's about enjoying this truly healthy way of living that results in weight loss and a healthy body (and mind!).

Your goal of losing weight will be best achieved with the help of natural supplements to ensure that your body is getting all the nutrients it needs. This is the best way to guarantee safe, healthy, and long term weight loss. As I have already mentioned in the introduction, all the natural tools I recommend in this book should be viewed as additional strategies. Nothing can replace a balanced diet and regular exercise, but the remedies I recommend not only do fit in, but they can also make the whole process a lot of easier and...more bearable! Your body will say *thank you!* I can promise you that.

If you have read this book because you want to lose weight, I suggest you make that commitment to a reliable fitness program and a healthy eating plan and to support it with one or several of the natural remedies mentioned in this book. Of course, don't take all of them at once.

If you enjoyed this book and would like to learn more about natural ways to lose weight, visit our blog for more tips and recipes:

www.HolisticWellnessProject.com

They all form part of my healthy weight loss tips series and are based on a balanced, alkaline diet, motivational factor as well as natural and holistic therapies to spice it up and achieve your weight loss goals faster!

I also hope that my books dedicated to weight loss treatments will also inspire you towards a healthy and balanced living. The unlimited energy levels and a vital, slim body will be the dessert that you deserve. It's not only about weight loss; first of all, it's about health!

If you enjoyed my book, it would be greatly appreciated if you left a review so others can receive the same benefits you have. Your review can help other people take this important step to take care of their health and inspire them to start a new chapter in their lives.

At the same time, <u>you can help me serve you and all my other readers</u> even more.

I'd be thrilled to hear from you!

Simply visit the link below or go <u>to your Amazon orders and write a short review</u> to share your experience. I know you are busy and I would like to thank you in advance for considering taking a couple of minutes to review this booklet.

Have a fantastic day,

I wish you all the best on your journey

Marta Tuchowska

www.HolisticWellnessProject.com

www.AlkalineDietLifestyle.com

Don't forget to grab your 3 free Alkaline Diet eBooks:

www.holisticwellnessproject.com/alkaline

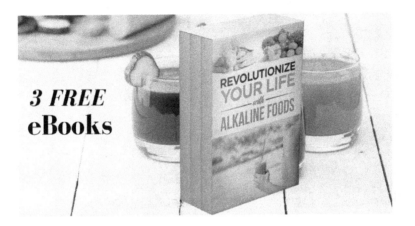

Marta's Wellness Books

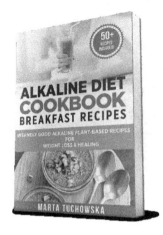

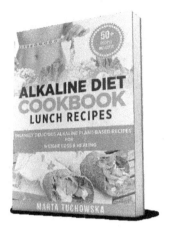

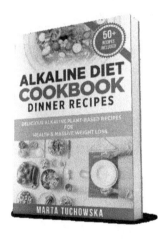

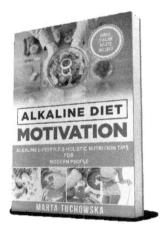

You will find more at:

www.holisticwellnessproject.com/alkaline-diet-books

www.holisticwellnessproject.com/books

Thanks again for your time and interest in my work.

It was a pleasure to "talk" to you,

I hope we "meet" again soon!

In the meantime, let's connect:

www.instagram.com/Marta_Wellness

www.facebook.com/HolisticWellnessProject

I wish you wellness, health, and success in whatever it is that you want to accomplish.

Marta

CPSIA information can be obtained
at www.ICGtesting.com
Printed in the USA
LVHW042235010920
664805LV00016B/329